Beat the Bloat – Saying Goodbye to Stomach Bloating Forever

Deb Maselli

Copyright © 2013 Deb Maselli

All rights reserved.

ISBN-13:978-1492707042

CONTENTS

Introduction	Pg# 5
Chapter One	Pg # 7
Chapter Two	Pg # 9
Chapter Three	Pg # 11
Chapter Four	Pg # 15
Chapter Five	Pg # 17
Chapter Six	Pg # 19
Chapter Seven	Pg # 21
Chapter Eight	Pg # 23
Chapter Nine	Pg # 27
Chapter Ten	Pg # 29
Chapter Eleven	Pg # 33

Introduction:

Unexplained bloating should always be evaluated by a medical professional to rule out serious medical conditions. Once you have been cleared by a doctor, you are free to assume you have the S.A.D. stomach. Otherwise known as, "the Standard American Diet stomach." As with any new program you are about to embark on, before taking any of the products recommended in the T.A.B. program, please check with your doctor. Some herbal supplements are not recommended to be taken with certain medications or medical conditions.
A healthy stomach usually feels like nothing. You should not be aware of your food being digested any more than you are aware of your elbow. But if you bloat after eating, you are very much aware of your stomach. You think about your stomach often during the day. You have all sorts of protocols to deal with it, and various pills and capsules rolling around in the bottom of your purse. After you eat, you wonder what people did before Lycra.
But really, the only thing you should notice after eating is that you are no longer hungry. If you experience stomach bloating after eating, your digestive system is out of balance.
Further, you should only be thinking about your bowels when you notice you need to have a bowel movement. This should happen at least once a day. When you feel the need for a bowel movement, you should have it, quickly and with no effort. You should be able to use a small piece of tissue to clean yourself.
When you have chronic gas, bloating and the occasional constipation that can come with it, it ends up running your life. **Think back to a time when you never thought about your stomach, except to notice that you were hungry. Let's get back to that time.**

Chapter One: How did we get here?

It's obvious to everybody that the standard American diet (the S.A.D.) is causing a tsunami of health problems. Obesity, diabetes, heart problems, chronic inflammation, vitamin and mineral deficiencies, GERD, skin eruptions and on and on are becoming the new normal of ill-health. But what nobody seems to be talking about is the gas and bloating the American diet causes. The S.A.D. doesn't just cause gas and bloating *while* you are eating it. It throws the digestive system out of balance, and the digestive system stays out of balance, until steps are taken to re-balance it.

Maybe nobody is talking about gas and bloating because it's not life threatening, or they think it's just a part of getting older. It may not be life threatening, but it is a serious quality of life issue that has little to do with age.

The American stomach is experiencing a slew of problems caused by the processed food in the Western diet. Now that the Western diet has been exported, people all over the world are experiencing the American uncomfortable stomach. Most American food companies are disingenuous at best. They see a trend and hop right on it. So, they think, Americans are becoming more concerned with health? No problem, slap on a label that touts added calcium or reduced fat or real juice, change the name from "cookies" to "breakfast bars" and who will know the difference?

Your stomach knows the difference. Most of the things a food a manufacturer will label as "healthy" I wouldn't feed to my dog. (And my dog will eat mushrooms in the yard and then throw up, so her standards are already pretty low.) That doesn't mean I'm for tighter regulations or that I don't sometimes eat junk. I live in the real world too and a lot of junk food tastes good and is really convenient. But, what it does mean is that I suffered unnecessarily for years before I figured out that the standard American diet was at the root of my digestive woes and what to do about it. I don't want you to suffer that long.

Pharmaceutical companies are perfectly delighted with our awful diet. I'm sure you know somebody on Prilosec. Everybody knows somebody on Prilosec. I used to be on Prilosec. I'm sure you've tried a number of over-the-counter products for relief. They do work to mask a symptom, but they don't work to fix the underlying problem. You may have tried probiotics, and then been disappointed when they didn't work. Or used Simethicone, in products like Gas-X. They're fine, but you have to keep taking them. And taking them. Of course, that's good business.

I discovered that throwing a remedy at only one aspect of an out-of-balance digestion doesn't work. Three components need to be addressed – Transit time, Absorption of nutrients and Bacteria re-establishment – T.A.B., for short. In the following chapters I'll explain digestive transit time, effective absorption of nutrients, friendly bacteria, how the T.A.B. program eliminates gas and bloating and provide you with information on nutrition to support your newly healed digestive system.

I won't suggest you give up all the foods you love. That's just not realistic. But I will give you the tools to repair your digestive system and, once repaired, how to add to the S.A.D. to encourage your body to thrive. The human body is geared to reach toward wellness. To return to a healthy state, all your digestive system requires is for you to provide the right environment.

Chapter Two: Digestive Transit Time

Transit time is how long your food takes to work its way through your digestive system and arrive in your toilet. This is a balancing act. Too fast, and you experience diarrhea. Too slow, and you're constipated. In general, the S.A.D. results in either constipation, or constipation with bouts of diarrhea. Interestingly, many people get so used to the bouts of diarrhea that when they don't have diarrhea they think all is well. They do not even realize that they are constipated. At that point, the digestive system has become unregulated and it is lurching forward and halting, and then lurching forward and halting, instead of moving forward smoothly and efficiently. Some people don't realize they are constipated because they have bowel movements on a regular schedule. But what's coming out may have been in their too long – the pipes are backed up.

It is noted in medical literature that a "normal" number of bowel movements for a healthy person can range from multiple times a day to three times a week. I don't happen to agree with three times a week. I believe a healthy digestion results in AT LEAST one bowel movement a day. It's important to keep the train moving. But the best predictor of your own normal schedule is how you feel. When your digestive system is sluggish, you feel sluggish and heavy and bloated. When your digestive system is in overdrive, you experience cramping, diarrhea and frequent trips to the bathroom. When your digestive system is working at an optimal level, you feel the need to have a bowel movement, go into the bathroom, are there for a short amount of time and then bounce out of the bathroom feeling light and comfortable.

Here are some guidelines on what you should be seeing in your toilet: (And you should be looking from time to time - what comes out is an accurate representation of what's going on in there.)

A Typical bowel movement is: fairly large, round and is brown or golden brown in color. It has a firm, but not hard or cracked, appearance. It should not float. You should have the bowel movement easily, without straining, and be able to clean yourself with a small piece of tissue. When you leave the bathroom you should feel lighter and have a sense of well-being.

A healthy bowel movement is not: dried out, pebbly, ribbon-like, watery, pale or green. (If you see red in your stool, have black, tarry stool, very pale stool or notice any sort of marked change in its appearance, see a medical professional to rule out serious causes.) If you're constipated, a bowel movement feels incomplete and your sense of relief, if you have it all, does not last long. If you are experiencing diarrhea, you feel better for a short amount of time and then the cycle starts again.

The T.A.B program brings digestive transit time into balance. Food moves through the digestive tract efficiently, extracting the nutrients a body needs to thrive, without hanging around too long and causing problems after it's served its purpose.

Chapter Three: Regulating Transit Time

The three digestive dynamos that regulate transit time are: Ginger, Magnesium and Psyllium seed husks.

Ginger is usually thought of as an old-fashioned remedy for upset stomachs. We all remember having ginger-ale for upset tummies as children. Ginger is highly effective for nausea, but that's not why it's a part of T.A.B. Ginger is also a powerful anti-inflammatory and does a remarkable job of regulating the transit speed of the digestive system. In T.A.B., Ginger is the conductor running the train.

Ginger is one of the most overlooked herbs. I believe people have the general impression that because it is a natural herb, it can't be strong enough for what ails them. That is not true. Ginger is powerful, can provide relief in minutes, is effective for calming Vagus nerve irritation (more about the Vagus nerve in Chapter Seven) and can protect from further bloating and gas for hours.

Would a glass of ginger-ale do all that for an unregulated digestive system? I doubt it. I suspect the amount of real ginger in a regular can of ginger-ale is miniscule and the added sugar won't be helpful. Diet ginger-ale may not have sugar, but many people with bloating find sugar substitutes particularly aggravating to their system. However, ginger powder is widely available in capsules. The standard capsule is 550mg and it can be taken on an empty stomach.

Magnesium is a mineral that delivers a big punch. Many Americans are deficient in magnesium and do not even know it. Magnesium deficiency is being worsened by processed food manufacturers who keep adding calcium into everything, but not pairing it with added magnesium. It has also been documented that people taking long-term doses of proton pump inhibitors like Nexium, Prevacid and Prilosec run the risk of low magnesium levels. If you notice that you are stiff and have muscle soreness in the morning or are prone to lower leg cramping, that's a good tip-off. In any event, adding magnesium at night will draw water into your colon, thereby making a bowel movement ever so much easier.

All magnesium types are not created equal. Some magnesium types are more bioavailable than others. Bioavailability simply means how well your body can use the particular nutrient. Some magnesium types, like magnesium oxide, are not highly available to your system. In general, if you buy the cheapest bottle of magnesium capsules you can find, you will get magnesium oxide. It WILL increase digestive transit time, in fact oxide is great at increasing transit time. But it may increase transit time too much, causing diarrhea. AND, your body will miss out on all the health benefits of magnesium in more bioavailable forms.

Research on magnesium is ongoing. It appears that magnesium plays a vital role in metabolism, cardiovascular health, regulating blood pressure, bone health and supporting the immune system. People who eat a diet primarily composed of non-processed whole grains, legumes and vegetables are probably not deficient in this mineral. Is that what you're eating? If not, your body would probably appreciate some extra magnesium.

Do not exceed 300 mg per day and look for a high quality blend. Use whatever magnesium blend works for you – just avoid a tablet that is comprised of ONLY oxide. Personally, I prefer Vital Nutrient's brand Triple Mag 250.

You will find that you have a personal schedule with magnesium. It is probably not necessary, or even beneficial, to take it every day. Once you have your digestive system back on track, you may find you only need to take it once or twice a week. Always take magnesium with food - ironically, it can be hard on an empty stomach.

Once you've got ginger driving the train and magnesium supplying the fluid, you need to give your digestive system something to work on. That's where psyllium seed husks comes in. This is especially important for people who snack on small meals all day or who take in less than twenty grams of fiber per day through their diet. Your digestive system will benefit from volume.

Many people with stomach bloating avoid adding extra fiber. It seems counter-intuitive to add bulk to a digestive system that already feels bloated. But bulk will stimulate peristalsis, the muscle contractions that will move the digested food through your system and into the toilet in a regular and comfortable manner, and that goes a long way to eliminate bloating. Psyllium seed husk is also a demulcent, so it will both soothe the intestinal tract while gently sweeping the intestines clean, carrying out bad bacteria and giving probiotics a better chance to take hold. About thirty percent of your stool is composed of dead bacteria. So, there's a lot of bacteria in there. It is also why, if your digestive system is working well, it seems like there's more coming out then you took in. Psyllium seed husks relieve both constipation and diarrhea by regulating transit time.

Chapter Four: Absorption of Nutrients

Absorption simply means how well the digestive tract is breaking down your food and absorbing the nutrients. When your digestive system is not breaking down and absorbing efficiently, you will experience bloating and gas. And, as if that isn't bad enough, when your digestive system is not breaking down food properly it languishes and ferments, resulting in smelly gas. For instance, gas that smells of sulfur is usually the result of improperly digested protein. Most people who are not properly breaking down their food begin to blame the food. They often make lists of 'trigger foods.' One day yogurt is fine, but now they decide they must be lactose intolerant because every time they eat yogurt, their stomach bloats like a balloon. Or, they may find that large amounts of protein result in rotten egg smelling gas. Or that their stomach is sticking out because they are retaining water, so salt is the problem. Or somebody told them that wheat is awful for digestion so it must be the sandwich they had for lunch. A person can spend years trying to figure out which foods are causing the problem. They begin to wonder why the list of things they can't eat keeps getting longer. But they will only find relief when they understand WHY, not WHAT.
The digestive system is out of balance and struggling to efficiently process food.
Unless you are actually allergic to a food item, you should be able to eat anything without experiencing gas and bloating. If you find you are in possession of an expanding list of foods you consider a problem, the answer isn't to eliminate the foods, the answer is to support the digestive system in breaking down the food.

Chapter Five: Digestive Enzymes

Your body spews digestive enzymes every time you eat. (At least, it's supposed to.) These enzymes break down and utilize the food that you have taken in. When enzymes are lacking, the breakdown is incomplete. This allows undigested food to travel through the digestive system, where it ferments. Supplementing with enzymes allows your body to utilize the food you eat and stop fermentation. This eliminates bloating and smelly gas.

Your body provides a wide array of enzymes from your mouth, your pancreas and your intestines. It is speculated that digestive enzymes decrease as we age. However, that doesn't explain why so many younger people are suffering from gas and bloating. My own feeling is that the S.A.D. in some way hastens the decrease in digestive enzymes or in some way suppresses them. This is pure speculation on my part and I don't have any scientific studies to back it up. But, I believe that the inflammatory nature of sugar is at the root of this problem. What I don't have to speculate on is the relief provided by digestive enzymes for gas and bloating.

If you are lacking in enzymes, it is very easy to confirm. Eat a problem food with an enzyme capsule. If you are deficient in enzymes you will have a completely different experience with that formerly problematic food. Suddenly, it's not a problem anymore. Reviews are mixed about taking digestive enzymes long term with every meal. Some people believe it is perfectly fine, others believe it will interfere with the body's own ability to generate enzymes. My own feeling is that enzymes do not need to be taken long term, with every meal. It is simply not necessary to use digestive enzymes in that way. My suggestion is to use the digestive enzymes as directed in the T.A.B. program for the seven days, and then use them only as needed. Once your digestive system is on its way to health, it will become clear to you where and when you need to use enzymes. For myself, in the beginning I took them with every major meal and also with yogurt, which was a particular problem for me. Now, I do not take them every day. I occasionally take them with a green smoothie in the morning, or when I decide to throw caution to the wind and eat a Big Mac, fries and a Coke, but even then not always. Let your body direct you. I have come to believe that once you are able to eliminate antacids and proton pump inhibitors from your life, acid levels in the stomach return to normal and enzymes quickly follow suit. Once your digestive system has been healed, it can more easily tolerate the occasional insults you pay it with the S.A.D., as long as you complement the S.A.D. with some real nutrition.

It is vital to use a reputable, and complete, enzyme supplement. Different enzymes process different types of food components. Read the label and make sure the enzymes you have chosen are plant based and contain the necessary enzymes to process protein, fat and carbohydrates. Though the directions may say to take two capsules with every meal, start with one capsule within thirty minutes of a largish meal or one capsule with a small meal that is the type of food you KNOW is a problem. The following is a sample of commonly available enzymes:

Lipase for fats
Amylase for carbohydrates
Protease for proteins

Most good brands also include other ingredients like papain and bromelain. Personally, I use GNC Super Digestive Enzymes. Papain chewable tablets are not as effective as a multi-enzyme, but they are great for digesting a meal that is primarily protein, are very inexpensive and are an easy supplement to have in your purse. Lactaid and other products designed to digest lactose are handy to have when you are just having a yogurt or glass of milk and taking a multi-enzyme would be over kill.

Again, you don't have to take enzymes forever. Once your digestive system begins to get back on track, you can, and should, ease off of them.

Chapter Six: Gut Bacteria

Your digestive system is a virtual zoo of friendly bacteria. Or, it should be. If you experience chronic bloating, it probably isn't. Whether it was caused by the S.A.D. or a course of antibiotics or stress or some other factor is irrelevant. An imbalance of helpful bacteria needs to be corrected, not just for how your stomach feels, but to ensure that your immune system is functioning at an optimal level. A good deal of your immune system resides in your gut. Fortunately, bacteria imbalance can be corrected. If you have tried **probiotics** in the past without noticeable relief, don't give up on them. In T.A.B. you'll be setting up the right circumstances for the friendly bacteria to take hold.

Supplemental probiotics are the live bacteria found in yogurts, capsules and elsewhere, meant to boost the helpful bacteria in your gut. There is some debate about whether probiotics do actually boost the number of good bacteria in the gut, or whether they just positively affect the expression of gut health. However, there is no debate that they are helpful in regulating the digestive system, whatever it is they are doing in there. Lactobacillus and Bifidobacteria are the most common strains associated with digestive health.

Now, these friendly bacteria are alive, and they need to eat. That brings us to prebiotics. Prebiotics feed the helpful bacteria you have just introduced, helping them thrive. Good sources of prebiotics are whole grains, almonds, honey and bananas (Though some people with an out of balance digestive system find bananas particularly difficult).

One of the nice things about a good quality yogurt is that a prebiotic is often included. Look for the words: Inulin, FOS, GOS or TOS.

This is particularly a good combination, since the probiotics and prebiotics are balanced. Vary the brands and types of yogurt, and look for low or no sugar. Read labels carefully – some yogurts are really a dessert and you might as well just have cookies. If you have not tried kefir yet, I would highly recommend it. It is a drinkable fermented milk product, not as sweet as yogurt, and is 99% lactose free. Lifeway kefir is turning up in more and more grocery stores. As an extra boost, keep a bottle of Lactobacillus chewable tablets on hand and take one with yogurt to take advantage of the prebiotic that has already been loaded into the product.

While it is vital to introduce good bacteria into a digestive system suffering from gas, bloating and constipation, it is just as vital to keep introducing it. Probiotics should be taken every day – think of them as a multi-vitamin for your stomach.

So, which probiotics will be most helpful to you? Start with a quality product from reputable manufacturer. At least guarantee yourself that what they say is in the package actually is. In particular, look for "live, active cultures" and a "use by" date. Large, reputable manufacturers have a lot to lose if they don't get it right, so they are less likely to cut corners and produce a shoddy product. Probiotics are one of those products that is extremely difficult to evaluate as a consumer. Unless you have your own lab, how would you know if the product actually contains enough live bacteria? It's not the time to bargain shop. From there, you may need to experiment with different strains – digestive environments are uniquely individual and what works well for one person may not be ideal for the next person. Be patient. If you have purchased a thirty-day supply, give it the whole thirty days to take effect. If the probiotic you have selected seems like it's not helping, move on to another strain. I particularly recommend Florastor for people who have tried probiotics in the past with little success. If you are brand new to probiotics, a thirty day starter pack, like Align, would be a good choice.

Chapter Seven: The Vagus Nerve

The vagus nerve is also called the "wandering nerve." It is long, and runs from your brain to your stomach. Many people with digestive problems, particularly gas, bloating and excessive acid, have an irritated vagus nerve. Irritation to the vagus nerve can also be caused by infections like h.pylori. Vagus nerve irritation is a big problem because the symptoms will not clue you in that it has anything at all to do with your digestion. Some people with an irritated vagus nerve experience heart pounding, racing or fluttering or a sense of dizziness. It can be frightening and someone experiencing this symptom can feel as if they are about to pass out. The difficulty is, these symptoms can be caused by much more serious issues. Anyone with an abnormal feeling in their chest, including pressure, rapid heartbeat, dizziness, any marked change or just an intuition that something is wrong should be evaluated by a medical professional immediately.
Many people with an irritated vagus nerve end up seeing a cardiologist. (And rightly so, these symptoms absolutely need to be evaluated by a medical professional) Should it be an irritated vagus nerve that is causing the symptoms, the person may sail through an echocardiogram, a stress test, getting wired for twenty-four hours – the whole drill. And the tests all come back fine. Once serious medical conditions are ruled out, the person may be told that they have experienced a panic attack, or perhaps they are swallowing too much air. Most medical professionals are not going to look for the connection between the vagus nerve and stomach issues.
The ingredient in T.A.B. that helps eliminate vagus nerve irritation is

ginger. It is a powerful anti-inflammatory and soothes the irritation. For people suffering from an irritated vagus nerve, ginger provides almost immediate relief and feels like a wonder drug.

Chapter Eight: Getting ready

You will need the following:

Psyllium seed husks
A Magnesium blend **not to exceed 300 mg**
Ginger in 550 mg **strength capsules**
Plant based multi-digestive enzymes
Florastor or the Probiotic of your choice

Please read the below tips before starting T.A.B.

1. **Magnesium and ginger.** If you tend toward bouts of diarrhea, limit your intake of magnesium to once or twice a week. If you tend toward constipation, take magnesium once a day until stools become a little loose and then adjust down until you find your optimum frequency. With ginger, be sure to wash the capsule all the way down – a half glass of water should be sufficient. Otherwise, you may feel a slight heat inside or be able to taste the ginger a bit. Personally, that doesn't bother me at all and I kind of like it in the winter time, but it's good to know about.

2. It is important to go slow. Your body does not like to be shocked and will not thank you for it. That's why the program is structured to build slowly. Example - there are thousands of people who will say they can't take psyllium because it gives them gas. Often, this is caused by using too much too soon. (I sympathize, I don't like to wait for anything either.) But DON'T do that. Start slow and easy with day one and go from there. Don't substantially change your diet.

Just eat what you normally would. You've probably been living with gas, bloating and constipation for a while, don't mess yourself up by being impatient.

3. Use the highest quality products you can afford. Once you are feeling better, you can start experimenting with lower cost options to see if you get the *same* relief. When experimenting with lower cost options, try just one new product at a time. That way, if you run into a problem and notice that you are slipping back into your old bloat cycle, you'll be able to pinpoint where you made the change. There is an exception to this - feel free to buy the cheapest psyllium husks you can find.

4. If you have been skipping around the book and haven't read the chapters on transit time, absorption and bacteria, please do so when you have the time. It's important to understand how the substances you will be taking work (and work synergistically together). Trying only one ingredient in the formula, rather than the whole formula together, may give you some relief, but not the complete relief you're looking for.

5. Notice that the Probiotics do not begin until day four. The first couple of days are designed to give you relief. You will feel better, begin moving out bad bacteria and your digestive system will calm down. Once your system feels better, then it's time to repair and get healthy again. As well, don't skip an ingredient because you've tried it in the past and it didn't work for you. These substances have a **synergistic effect when taken to together**. This program isn't meant to cover up a symptom, it's meant to heal from ingestion to toilet, from digestive dis-ease to digestive health.

6. Convenience. Gather all your products together and divide them up into a week's worth of Ziploc snack bags and label them by day. That way, you can just throw them into your bag, ready to go, without dragging around pill bottles and constantly going back to the directions.

7. This is not a forever program. Listen to your body. It will tell you which supplements you can ease off of and when. For instance, you may find that you only need the enzymes when eating a large amount of protein, or that you only need magnesium once a week, etc. You may repair your gut to the point that you don't need anything at all. Then, the next time you have a course of antibiotics or spend an entire weekend eating pizza and you slip back to square one - you'll know what to do about it.

8. This is totally obvious but bears repeating - drink enough water and move around. Water is the grease your intestines will use to slide waste down the tubes, rather than sitting where it is, stagnating and fermenting. Moving around doesn't mean violent exercise. Walking around after eating is sufficient to move things along.

9. Before trying any new supplement always talk to your doctor. Some herbs are contraindicated for certain medications and conditions. For example, ginger has blood thinning properties and should not be taken by people who are already taking a blood thinning medication or who have a bleeding disorder. Again, your own physician will know best if a product may be harmful for you.

Chapter Nine: The T.A.B. Program

Day One:
1 ginger capsule on an empty stomach, first thing in the morning
1 enzyme capsule and 1 ginger capsule with each substantial meal
1 enzyme capsule with any smaller meal that contains a problem food
1 magnesium capsule in the evening, with food
1/2 teaspoon psyllium husk mixed with 8 ounces of water, taken at any time

Day Two:
1 ginger capsule on an empty stomach, first thing in the morning
1 enzyme capsule and 1 ginger capsule with each substantial meal
1 enzyme capsule with any smaller meal that contains a problem food
1 magnesium capsule in the evening, with food
1 teaspoon psyllium husk mixed with 8 ounces of water, taken at any time

Day Three:
1 ginger capsule on an empty stomach, first thing in the morning
1 enzyme capsule and 1 ginger capsule with each substantial meal
1 enzyme capsule with any smaller meal that contains a problem food
1 magnesium capsule in the evening, with food
1 and 1/2 teaspoon psyllium husk mixed with 8 ounces of water, taken at any time.

Day Four:
1 ginger capsule on an empty stomach, first thing in the morning

1 enzyme capsule and 1 ginger capsule with each substantial meal
1 enzyme capsule with any smaller meal that contains a problem food
1 magnesium capsule in the evening, with food
1 Tablespoon psyllium husk mixed with 8 ounces of water, taken at any time.
Probiotics, as directed by the manufacturer.

Day Five:
1 ginger capsule on an empty stomach, first thing in the morning
1 enzyme capsule and 1 ginger capsule with each substantial meal
1 enzyme capsule with any smaller meal that contains a problem food
1 magnesium capsule in the evening, with food
1 and 1/2 tablespoons psyllium husk mixed with 16 ounces of water, divided into two servings and taken at different times of day
Probiotics, as directed by the manufacturer.

Day Six:
1 ginger capsule on an empty stomach, first thing in the morning
1 enzyme capsule and 1 ginger capsule with each substantial meal
1 enzyme capsule with any smaller meal that contains a problem food
1 magnesium capsule in the evening, with food
2 tablespoons psyllium husk mixed with 16 ounces of water, divided into two servings and taken at different times of day
Probiotics, as directed by the manufacturer

Day Seven:
1 ginger capsule on an empty stomach, first thing in the morning
1 enzyme capsule and 1 ginger capsule with each substantial meal.
1 enzyme capsule with any smaller meal that contains a problem food
1 magnesium capsule in the evening, with food
2 and 1/2 tablespoons psyllium husk mixed with 16 ounces of water, divided into two servings and taken at different times of day
Probiotics, as directed by the manufacturer

Hopefully, you're feeling better now. Time to begin supporting your digestive system and working toward health. I won't advocate giving up all the junk food you love, but you do need to add good nutrition.

Chapter Ten: Rebuilding healthy digestion

It would be great if you would confine yourself to eating only healthy, non-processed foods. (It would be great if I did that, too.) On the off chance you are not going to do that, at least feed your body once a day with something it can really appreciate.
Green smoothies are an easy way to feed your body with a plethora of micronutrients. You might hate the taste of kale or Swiss chard or spinach, but a well-made green smoothie makes it possible to take in all these nutrient-rich foods without tasting them.

My green drink recipe: All of the ingredients do something in particular. If made according to the following recipe, it will have an apple-lemony flavor. (Calories: about 160   Fat: 6 grams of good fat and 0 grams of bad fat)
The dark, green leafy vegetables supply your body with vitamins and nutrients, particularly things you are probably not getting elsewhere, like vitamin K.
Lemon is a tried and true digestive supporter, will help your body release excess water, and the skin is full of powerhouse bio-flavanoids.
Granny Smith apples are great soluble fiber and are loaded with vitamin C. They have a bold enough flavor to override the taste of the greens.
Chia seeds are an excellent source of protein and omega-3, do not need to be ground up like flax seeds, and act as a thickener to the drink.
Powdered greens – concentrated greens will supercharge the drink with mega-dense nutrients.

Avocado - this small amount of good fat is good for you and gives the drink a filling and rich, creamy consistency.

Green drink:
1C Swiss chard or other dark green leafy vegetable
1 thick slice of lemon with skin
1/2 granny smith apple with skin, seeds removed
1T chia seeds
1 t powdered greens
1/8th of an avocado (about 1T)
If you are using a Nutribullet, pack everything down into the larger cup and add water to the maximum fill line

It's important to rotate greens. Different types of greens will not affect the taste of the drink, except for the most bitter, like mustard greens and arugula. Greens like kale, spinach, collard greens and bok choy are super-nutritious, but if eaten every single day in large quantities they can affect metabolism in susceptible individuals. Rather than try to remember which green belongs to which family, just buy something different every time you shop. That will give your body a smorgasbord of nutrients that it has been looking for and not finding in the S.A.D.

Nutribullet - I recommend the Nutribullet (not the plain old Magic Bullet, they are totally different) for a whole host of reasons. The Nutribullet is easy to use, it's easy to clean, it has a powerful motor, and the blending cups have twist on lids, turning them into to-go cups. It's very convenient to add everything together in the large blender cup and stick it in the fridge overnight. In the morning, just add water, blend and go. Whatever you decide to use – don't choose a juicer. It removes all the fiber and it's a real pain to use and keep clean. (I have one, it's in my closet.)

Greens Boxes - These plastic boxes extend the life of your veggies and keep them crisp and fresh. There's nothing worse than greens that have gone slimy in the vegetable drawer. I generally buy greens once a week, clean them, trim off large stalks, let them dry and load them into the green boxes. Then, they are ready to go for the week.

Flavor - the above recipe tastes apple-lemony. Once you have the base - greens, 1/8 avocado, 1T chia, you can flavor it however you like. I use the above recipe because I find it most compatible with the base. Some powdered greens supplements are on the bitter side, so if you are brand new to green smoothies, leave them out for a week or so and then add them in tiny amounts until your taste buds become accustomed to them.

You can also make any sort of fruit smoothie in the **Nutribullet**, but I don't. It's a huge amount of sugar and you will miss all the great nutrients from greens. Some people are not so much concerned with the flavor as with the color. If that bothers you, put the smoothie in an opaque travel mug with a lid so you don't actually see it. The drink may seem strange at first, but it will quickly grow on you because it will make your body feel good.

Going forward - As you become more aware of the nutrients you are taking in, you can expand what you are adding to your green smoothie. There are hundreds of books filled with recipes for green smoothies if you find you don't have your own ideas. Your smoothies should be personalized to fill the holes in your diet. In the meantime, if you have been subsisting on the S.A.D., your body will find the basic green smoothie a virtual fiesta of nutrition.

Chapter Eleven: Further Supplementation

The TA.B. regimen will get your digestive system back on track. However, it's always helpful to have more in your digestive arsenal for when particular problems or unexpected situations crop up. You may feel great day to day, but then a vacation trip seems to throw things off. Below is a list of helpful products for unexpected symptoms. As always, talk your doctor before adding any supplement.

Activated Charcoal – activated charcoal helps with absorbing intestinal gas and reducing smell.

Chlorophyll – chlorophyll capsules 'sanitize' your digestive tract, reducing smell.

The Republic of Tea "Get relief" is a yummy, minty blend that is helpful for stomach gas.

Triphala - an age-old Ayurvedic herbal blend used to support the digestive system.

Glucomannan – this powder is made from the konjac root. It is an excellent source of fiber and gives the stomach a full feeling. It may be helpful for weight loss for that reason. Glucomannan capsules must be taken with a full glass of water since they expand rapidly.

dgl– dgl is an herbal extract that soothes the digestive tract by increasing the mucous coating in the digestive system.

Colostrum – **colostrum** supports the friendly bacteria in your gut.

Aloe Vera juice – drinkable aloe vera coats the digestive tract.

Slippery elm tea – slippery elm is soothing and coats the digestive tract.

Kefir – kefir is an excellent substitute for yogurt, as it is 99% lactose free.

The Republic of Tea - "Get Probiotic" is a tea enhanced by the probiotic ganeden BC.

And finally, life is meant to be lived. There is so much to do and see and think about. There is also so much junk food to eat. Moderation and treating your digestive system kindly will pay you back a thousand fold. I hope you are able to go forward, feeling truly alive and bursting

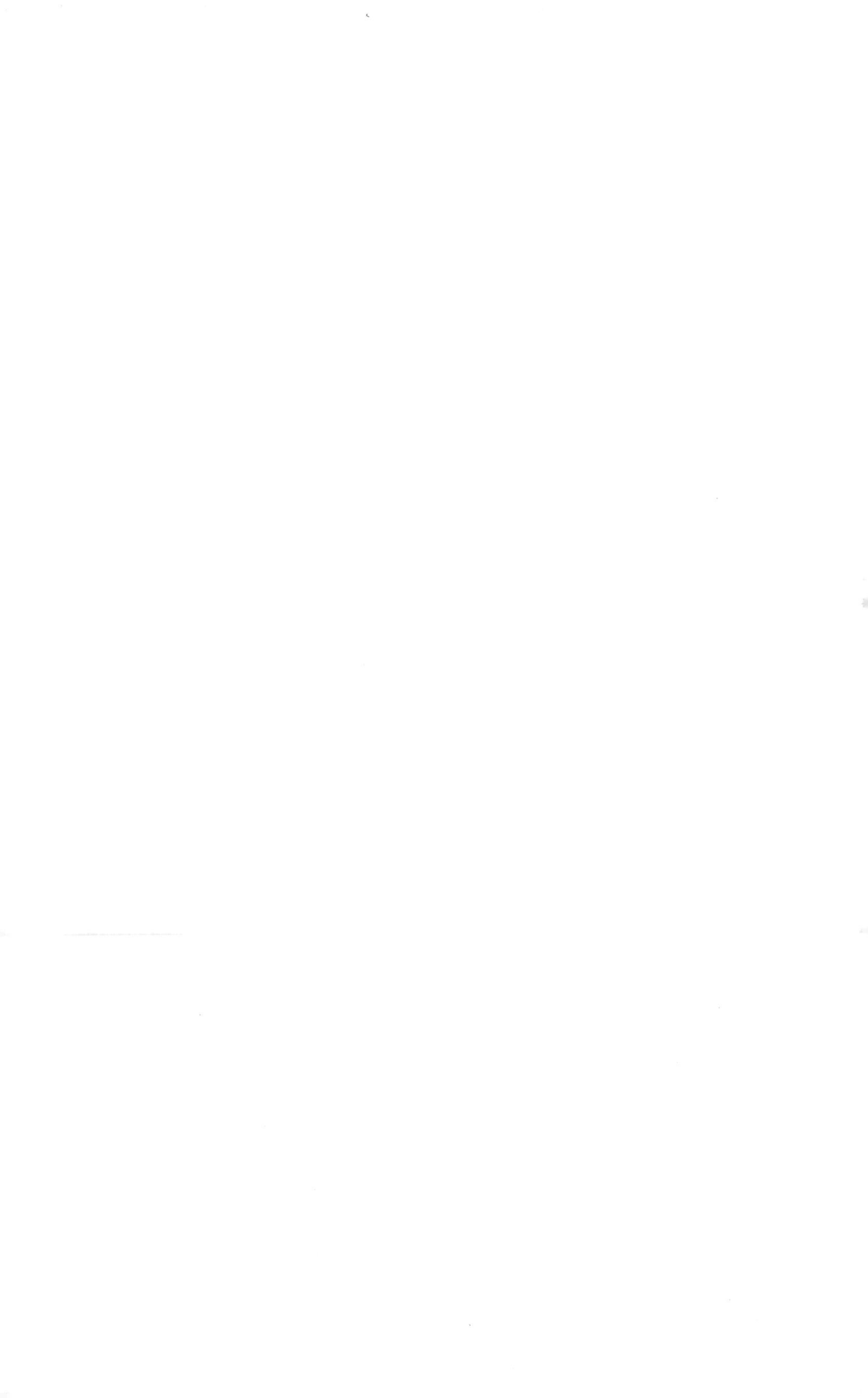

Printed in Great Britain
by Amazon